CW00523360

The wellness diet: how to lose weight quickly while staying healthy

Luca Cutrone

2

The Wellness Diet ©2020 - Luca Cutrone

"This is my advice

if you insist on losing weight:

eat as much as you like,

just don't swallow."

Harry Secombe

6

Disclaimer

This book is provided for the unic purpose of providing relevant information on a specific topic for which every reasonable effort has been made to ensure that it is accurate and reasonable.

This volume contains food information based on the author's experience. They are in no case intended as a substitute for a diet prescribed by a dietician. There are no guarantees of success: the author assumes no responsibility for desired results not fully achieved.

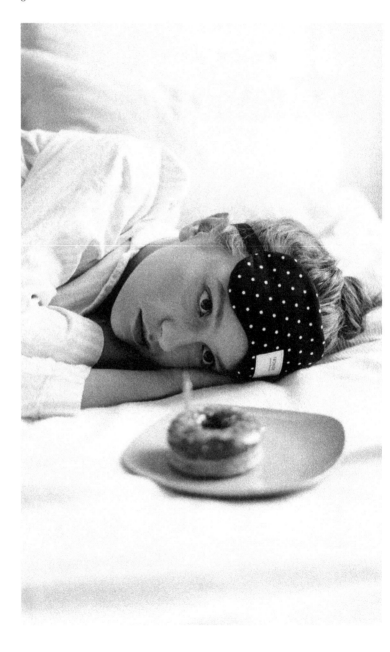

Summary

10

Introduction

I want to lose weight quickly.

Few other phrases we have repeated more often than this one. Two kilos, twenty kilos... for the summer and the costume rehearsal, for the imperfections...but is it possible to do it while staying healthy? That's what I will try to explain in this volume, starting from my personal knowledge and experience.

I've been practicing kick-boxing at a competitive level since I was 11 years old. I have an experience of about 120 matches between amateurs and professionals, I won twice the 67kg Italian title. Now I've retired, and I currently teach in two gyms in Novara. Nutrition, both in the "cruising" phase and in the preparation for the match, has been an element that I have always held in great consideration.

To this experience in the field I then added, after a few years of work, my university studies. The degree in food science has provided me with a whole series of tools and knowledge to deal with the chapter nutrition in much more scientific terms, making me discover in detail all those biochemical reactions of which before I had just a smattering or a vague hint.

Then the bad thing happened. In 2009 I suffered a heavy knee injury that forced me to an operation and rehabilitation. Months and months away from the ring and the gym: it was my greatest passion, and I suffered a lot. To this was added family and work problems, as well as an important mourning. So I went through a period of great stress. For almost a year I didn't train and I literally stuffed myself with junk food and junk food, rising from about 70 to almost 90 kilos.

Then, one day, I looked in the mirror and realized that that wasn't me.

I ended up embodying everything I had always hated. Enough. It was time to change. It was time to go on a diet.

But what kind of diet? I knew that a tight low carb would require a degree of sacrifice that I was unable to withstand at the time, and that the risk of relapse from that type of diet was high anyway. So I tried to mediate what was my knowledge with a type of diet that was not a devastating sacrifice but one that would guarantee constancy, and to help me with the various stratagems useful to fight the real enemy of every person who goes on a diet: HUNGER.

PHYSIOLOGY OF SLIMMING

Let's start with some basic concepts.

First: not everything is possible. We cannot lose twenty/thirty kilos in a month of course. Impossible.

One kilo of fat in our body is about 7000 calories. How come 7000 and not 9000, since one gram of fat is about nine calories? Simple: in the adipocyte (a connective tissue cell whose function is to synthesize, accumulate and release lipids) water is bound to lipids. So the real calorie content of our fat is not 9000 calories, but 7000.

This explains why, in the first week of diet, we lose a lot of weight: we are actually losing water, not fat, water that was linked to our glycogen reserves.

After ten to fifteen days the excess fat water is almost totally lost and you start to burn the excess fat... and in fact the slimming slows down considerably.

Second: you can never burn ONLY fat. This will sadden most people as it saddened me the first time we studied the subject during the years of university. Together with fat loss, in fact, there is always a loss of muscle mass, but this loss can be amortized or contained in various ways that I will explain later. One method to understand if they are burning fat or muscle mass is to take the *circumferences*: precisely of the waist, thighs and hips when we want to measure fat, forearms and calves to verify that there is not excessive loss of muscle mass.

Third: Physiologically, we can lose at most one and a half percent of our body weight per week. Here is the second reason why our weight loss will be more and more dampened, that is a pure matter of percentage: if we weigh 100 kilos we can lose 1 kilo per week, when we reach 90 we will lose 0.9, 80 0.8 and so on. Beyond these values we are SURELY burning lean mass too, which we should avoid as much as possible (as far as possible).

Fourth: the advice in this volume is aimed at people who consume at least 28 calories per kilo of body weight (men) and 26 calories per kilo of body weight (women). Those who do not take these minimum calorie values are probably eating too little, and should therefore avoid thinking about a slimming diet, let alone a fast one.

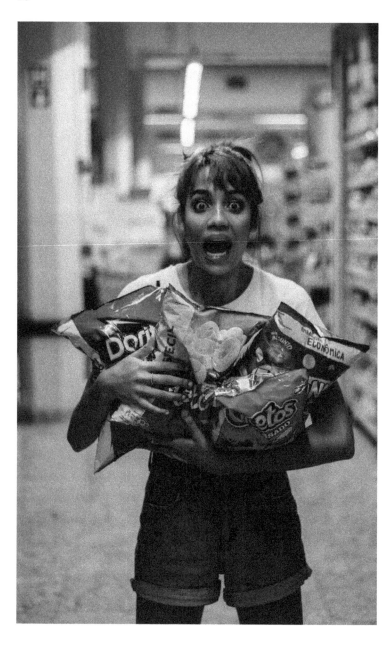

WHY FATTENING

Many people are looking for a specific culprit for their lack of weight loss. How many times have you heard guys complaining about blaming carbohydrates, hormones, slow metabolism "of nature"?

Well, bullshits.

Do carbohydrates make you fat?

Due also to the various low-carb diets, the first to end up in the dock are carbohydrates. Carbohydrates are the nutrients that provide clean energy (if we use protein for energy purposes we "dirty" the body with nitrogenous waste) and immediate (it takes longer to dismantle fats). We know eating sugars blocks lipolysis, i.e. the breakdown and burning of fats. The body stops burning fat and starts burning carbohydrates. It is therefore obvious that a higher dose than the ideal individual carbohydrate intake, depending on lifestyle and energy needs, tends to keep body fat intact. It is therefore not the carbohydrates themselves that become fat, but act as a "preservative".

Lipids make you fat?

Fats, unlike what is thought, perform different functions: an energetic function, a structural one, a vitamin one, an essential one and a reserve one. The latter type is the one often under accusation: actually, they go to compose the energy reserves for the "lean periods" that in ancient times, at the beginning of evolution, could last even longer. There was not a breakfast, a lunch and a dinner. It was hunted and collected when the opportunity arose: part of that energy had to be stored. However, it should be noted that if the balance between ingested fat and fat transformed into Acetyl Coenzyme A (as a result of beta-oxidation) translates into energy production (ATP) there is no problem. The problem arises when there is an excess of calories: then the Acetyl Coa is converted into fat. So it's not the lipids themselves that make you fat.

Do proteins make you fat?

Proteins are the macronutrient with the highest thermogenic effect, i.e. they require a higher Specific Dynamic Action. About a quarter of the calories introduced with protein are burned to digest the protein itself. In addition, proteins help our body to direct nutrients to muscle tissue and not fat tissue. Finally they have a high satiating power.

Do hormones make you fat?

Many times it has been heard that insulin is the cause of loss of weight. This is partially true: insulin regulates blood glucose levels by reducing blood glucose through the activation of different metabolic and cellular processes, and is responsible for the process of lipogenesis, i.e. the storage of lipids within the adipose tissue. A high level of insulin induces a sense of satiety, a low level of insulin (as in diabetics or obese people) does not block the stimulus of hunger and induces to eat more. However, the stimulation of insulin is given by the amount of carbohydrates we introduce, their glycemic load and the energy intake of the day. And we return to the question of "calorie deficit", i.e. ingesting fewer calories than our daily needs.

After having debunked some myths and made some clarity, we then enter the "hot" zone, the core of the matter. We start with some general indications, a memorandum of concepts always useful, and then we will analyze each aspect more specifically.

Finally we will show a practical example.

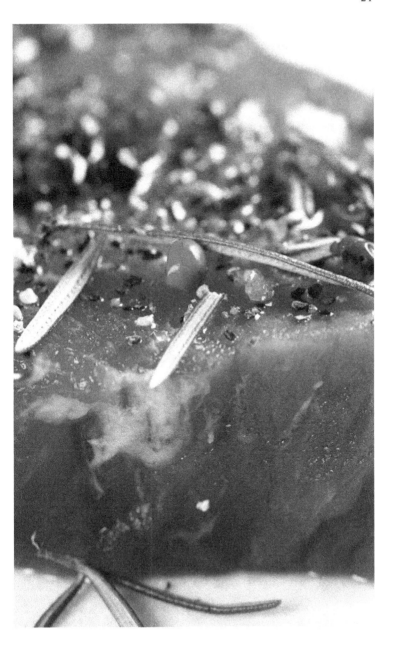

GENERAL INDICATIONS

1   TAKE A GOOD PROTEIN SHARE

A macronutrient that is never spared is protein. Proteins are the main "conservative agent" of lean mass and are at the same time a powerful filler.

2   TAKE A GOOD AMOUNT OF FIBER

An optimal amount of fiber is essential, we are talking about 30 grams per day. In addition to regulating the intestinal transit, they also help with the sense of satiety.

3   DRINK A LOT OF WATER

There's a tendency in many people who take in insufficient water to exchange the thirst for hunger. Drinking during the day, both water and herbal teas (not carbonated or sweetened drinks) helps to fill the stomach and feel less hungry. The ideal amount should be at least 30 deciliters per 10 kilos of weight.

4   USE CONDIMENTS SPARINGLY

You must have heard this too many times, but it's really important: you often don't notice the amount of butter, oil or anything else that you add to a food, which by its nature may not be very caloric, but in this way it becomes so. As a general indication, prefer oil to other seasonings and use a quality extra virgin olive oil. But always in moderation!

5   VEGETABLES IN ALL MAIN DISHES

Vegetables are also an excellent filler and are rich in mineral salts and vitamins. Better raw than cooked, because with cooking there's an important dispersion of vitamins.

6 WHOLE SUGARS INSTEAD OF REFINED SUGARS

Even this consideration is now quite well known: whole grains have undergone fewer industrial processing processes, are therefore potentially more "healthy", have a greater quantity of fiber and give a greater sense of satiety. For a palate accustomed to eating refined bread and pasta at first it will be a bit 'difficult to get used to, but your body will thank you.

7 PREFER FISH AND WHITE MEAT TO RED MEAT

In addition to a purely caloric speech, fish (especially blue) is less subjected to external agents such as antibiotics and pollutants (except mercury for large fish).

8 DO NOT IDLE AT HOME

The house is the realm of temptations and distractions. To waste time, to waste time, to be trifled with, not to engage in anything active means to increase the risk of opening the refrigerator and doing that outrage, which then become two, which become three and so on. Stay as active as possible, go out, or if you stay at home try to engage with something and do not stay on the couch watching TV.

9 MANAGE MEALS ACCORDING TO YOUR INCLINATIONS

Contrary to what many people think, there are no strict rules on the number of meals per day: the ideal would be to make from two to five, depending on one's "psychological needs", that is the necessary to suffer as little hunger as possible.

10 MOVEMENT

Training, unfortunately for lazybones, is essential: intense physical activity for a sufficient number of times a week (at least three) combined with a dynamic lifestyle in itself (e.g. walking or cycling instead of driving when possible) burn calories, increase muscle mass and reactivate the metabolism.

PROTEINE

We have already said that a macronutrient should never be missing from the diet is protein. Why?

First of all, proteins are formed by the union of simpler molecules, called amino-acids, which combine with each other through peptide bonds. In human body there are about 50,000 protein molecules whose function is determined by their amino acid sequence.

The chemical structure of protein amino-acids is composed of the carbon atom to which they are bound:

- a carboxylic group
- an amine group
- one atom of hydrogen
- a side chain or group R

They are divided into simple protein (composed exclusively of amino-acids) and conjugated protein (also composed of other chemical elements).

Since they are subject to deterioration, they are continuously disposed of and replaced by new proteins, in a process known as *protein turnover*. The amount of protein subject to protein *turnover on a* daily basis is about 4 grams per kg of body weight. Just a small part of this is lost and it's necessary to recover it through nutrition: in adults, we talk about 30-40 g of protein per day, a value that seems minimal, but if not restored can have serious consequences on body composition and health. In a state of protein deficiency, in fact, the body will affect the reserves present in the muscles, with a decrease in muscle mass and physical performance: if this process is maintained over time, the risk is that of deterioration and malnutrition. The introduction of proteins with food is also necessary because the body cannot synthesize 8 of the 20 amino-acids it needs to build proteins: these are called essential amino-acids.

PROTEIN FUNCTIONS

Let's see briefly what proteins are used for, their use within the body.

CONTRACTING FUNCTION: proteins within the muscle (myosin and actin) are responsible for the contraction function following a neurological stimulus. Bend an arm, lift a leg, run...

REGULATORY FUNCTION: proteins are used to regulate certain chemical processes, such as insulin.

TRANSPORT FUNCTION: the proteins inside the blood vessels carry various chemical elements. Hemoglobin, for example, carries oxygen, while lipoproteins carry lipids (fats).

ENZYMATIC FUNCTION: some proteins, such as catalase, ribonuclease, phosphofructokinase and trypsin act as accelerators for some biological reactions.

IMMUNITARY FUNCTION: immunoglobulins, i.e. globular proteins involved in the immune response.

Proteins are fundamental for *structural* reasons, but they are also the least efficient fuel to produce energy compared to carbohydrates and fats, as well as producing a lot of waste: the body will transform proteins into fuel only in the absence of the other two macronutrients. This is, to make a long story short, what all diets with very high protein content and very low carbohydrate and fat content are aiming at: this type of diet, however, does not consider the fact that 1) the kidney load actually becomes important 2) it is UNAVOIDABLE, with this system, to go and attack even the lean mass.

But let's leave this element out for now. Let's start by saying that, despite the demonization (and sometimes the mystification) suffered by proteins, especially animal proteins, in recent years, sometimes for "noble causes", for example with regard to the speech of intensive farming and environmental issues, proteins are a fundamental component at the structural level of our body.

Why are they considered so important in a diet? Let's now analyze some of the peculiarities of proteins that differentiate them from other macronutrients.

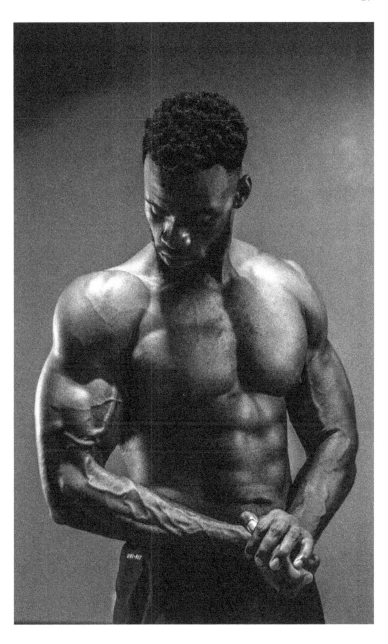

MUSCLE STRUCTURE

It's often said that "muscles are made up of proteins", or that proteins are the majority component of muscle. Let's shake on a myth. The muscles are composed of:

- ✓ Water (75%)
- ✓ protein (16-20%)
- ✓ lipids (3-7%)
- ✓ glycogen (1%)
- ✓

In addition, to a lesser extent, other components such as creatine and phosphates.

We also specify that there are three types of muscle:

- ✓ smooth muscle (present in the viscera and large blood vessels)
- ✓ heart muscle (heart)
- ✓ skeletal muscle (those related to the skeleton and therefore to movement)

The first two are the *involuntary* muscles: moved by an automatism of the body. The skeletal muscle is instead the set of voluntary muscles, i.e. responding to a nervous stimulus that starts by the will of the individual.

The protein income goes to preserve muscle mass from auto-cannibalism that could result from the shortage (as explained with regard to protein turnover), also increasing muscle volume increases basal metabolism (the share of calories burned to maintain simple body functions), thus directly affecting the decrease in fat mass in favor of lean.

T.I.D.

One of the main factors to consider, as far as the dietary potential of proteins is concerned, is undoubtedly the T.I.D., i.e. *Thermogenesis induced by diet.* What does it mean?

All macronutrients (carbohydrates, fats, proteins) must be broken down, digested, to be absorbed by the bloodstream and go to perform their functions. The digestion itself requires a certain amount of energy, therefore calories: this is thermogenesis.

Each nutrient has a different T.I.D. index:

- ✓ fats: 2%
- ✓ carbohydrates: 5%
- ✓ proteins: 25%

Therefore, taking 100g of tuna, with a total amount of protein of 25 g and an energy value of 4kcal for each gram of protein, we will use only to digest this tuna 25kcal, that's a quarter of the total calories ingested. Convenient, right?

SENSE OF SATIETY

Another very important element to consider is the ability of proteins to stimulate the sense of satiety. It may seem like something needless, but it's essential to be able to carry on a diet without unnecessary suffering (and without throwing in the towel).

We can classify the sense of satiety in two categories: short term sense of *satiation, which is* what develops while you are eating or immediately afterward, and long term sense of satiety, which refers to the hours after the last meal.

There're about 20 hormones operating in those parts of the brain where the appetite and satiety receptors are located. In particular, three of them stimulate satiety either indirectly, through the nerves leading to the brain, or directly through blood vessels.

-When food fills the stomach, especially bulky food rich in water, it stimulates the pancreas to produce a hormone called PP, which gives a sense of satiety for a few hours.

-When proteins and fats are consumed, cholecystokinin (CCK) is released in the duodenum, which signals the brain to stop eating: this explains why both fats and proteins have a satiating effect greater than carbohydrates.

-In the cells of the intestinal mucosa of the ileum and colon, proteins stimulate the production of another hormone: Peptide YY (PYYY), which is active after an hour or two after a meal and remains high for about six hours, limiting the onset of appetite.

So proteins produce both short-term and long-term satiety.

PARTITIONING

Energy partitioning is the use of our calories ingested in different energy substrates: for instance, where does what we eat end up, whether in adipose or muscle tissue. In a diet, of course, we are interested in increasing muscle tissue and decreasing fat tissue.

Partitioning is influenced by several factors:

- **genetic** (on which we can not intervene)
- **hormonal structure** (on which we can intervene but in a very limited way, for example with more regular sleep/wake hours)
- **power supply** (on which, obviously, we can intervene)

And here is the salient point: a high protein meal is able to better convey the caloric intake to the muscle tissue and not the adipose one, while protecting the lean mass from the consumption caused by a low-calorie regime.

WHICH PROTEINS TO TAKE?

There has been for a long time, and is still ongoing, a debate on which type of protein is best used. Let's try to make some clarity on the subject.

VEGETABLE OR ANIMAL PROTEINS?

The first aspect of this "bitter debate" about proteins concerns the concept of the vegetal/animal. Here not only the discourse of the nutritional value of protein itself is intersected, but also a series of ethical concepts that, although respectable and sharable, have little to do with the purely dietary discourse: this is the case of those who support a vegan diet as the best possible and the closest to the primeval nature of man (not to mention further and more drastic derivatives such as raw food or fruitarianism).

Now: without pretending to have the truth in our pockets and without making propaganda for or against, it must be recognized that most studies tend to consider the introduction of animal proteins in our diet a *fundamental* step in our evolution, something that has contributed to increase the brain and physical faculties of man and make him the homo-sapiens that we all know today.

Said that, are vegetable or animal proteins better? From a purely nutritional point of view, there is little difference between the two: both are, at the end of the fair, amino acid chains. From the point of view of their biological value, i.e. the presence of essential amino acids, the more a food has a composition similar to the human one, the higher will be its value: from this point of view, the value of animal proteins is slightly higher than vegetable ones, because animal proteins present the complete amino acid picture (all essential amino acids are present) while in vegetable proteins there is the so called *limiting* amino acid, i.e. missing (or present in very low doses) that affects the protein synthesis of the others. Another "disadvantageous" factor is the presence of other nutrients that slow down the assimilation of plant proteins. Finally, the vegetable sources with greater presence of protein, such as legumes, also have a significant amount of carbohydrates: for example, on 100 grams of beans I have 20 grams of protein and the rest are almost exclusively carbohydrates.

Obviously, the discussion on the QUALITY of animal proteins remains open: there is no doubt that certain foods should be avoided, such as preserved meat, sliced meats, sausages, rich in fat and preservatives; overcooked and burnt red meat that can be toxic; and instead to prefer fish such as blue fish, perhaps steamed.

PROTEIN POWDER?

Although the consumption of protein powder is increasing strongly, there is a generalized veil of distrust. Are you motivated?

Let's say it now: NO. The protein intake is very important because, as already explained, proteins are the building blocks of our body. Especially those who do sport need to increase the protein intake, causing the continuous breaking of muscle fiber and therefore the necessary repair.

So protein supplements do nothing but increase your protein intake WITHOUT needing to eat more and therefore also take other fats, other carbohydrates, other calories.

In particular, whey proteins seem to be ideal: in addition to the effects on muscle mass they also have beneficial effects on the body and nervous system.

They are marketed in three forms: concentrated, isolated and hydrolyzed. The difference is in the speed of absorption, which goes in ascending order. Preferably it is better to take them after physical activity, as the body is more receptive and therefore the repaired tissues will be specifically those broken during training.

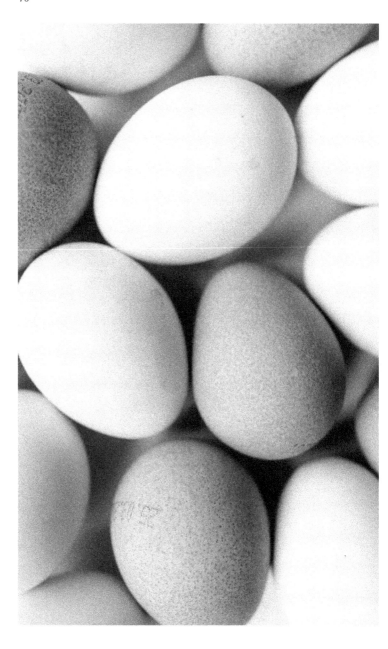

FIBERS

Fibers are very important in our diet.

In order to understand the topic well we start from the intestinal villi, the cells that make up our intestines. They continue the digestion that begins in the mouth and then in the stomach; they must then be able to recognize the various nutrients the various molecules; prevent the entry of toxic and harmful substances into the bloodstream and finally absorb nutrients. So, it can be said that our health goes from good intestinal health. The primary form of sustenance comes from the medium and short chain saturated fatty acids of the food we eat (to be precise acetic acid, proprioonic acid and butyric acid) but more easily these come from the enterocytes thanks to the digestion of intestinal bacteria, which are able to break them down and transform them into short chain fatty acids by coming into contact with certain types of dietary fiber. Fiber thus becomes the main nutrient for our enterocytes. A healthy enterocyte also sends signals to our satiated brain: therefore it is much easier to realize that we are satiated when our intestinal cells are well rather than when we eat low quality food and do not realize that we are introducing too much energy compared to our caloric needs. For example: whole grains (with the same number of calories) do not make you lose more weight than refined ones but give you a greater sense of satiety and therefore eat less, as well as a better quality of food due to less processing.

It's also necessary to be careful not to come into contact with too many harmful substances: for example, if we eat too much meat, especially if processed, putrefactive processes take place in our intestines. Fibers also in this case speed up the passage of these substances in the intestine and the enterocytes are not in contact with these harmful substances; other types of fibers are able to incorporate and isolate them. There is a direct correlation between health and protection of intestinal cells compared to the amount of fiber we eat.

Finally the fibers also have a positive effect on cholesterol levels, especially the bad cholesterol the way. The body degrades cholesterol through the secretion of bile juice: the fibers chelate the bile salts and do not allow normal reabsorption by the body.

Recommended levels of dietary fiber are around 30 grams per day. It is not ideal to eat less or eat more, which could lead to constipation and irritation of the intestine. The classic foods richer in fiber are oat bran or wheat bran, which can be taken through cereals or directly to teaspoons, perhaps mixed in yogurt.

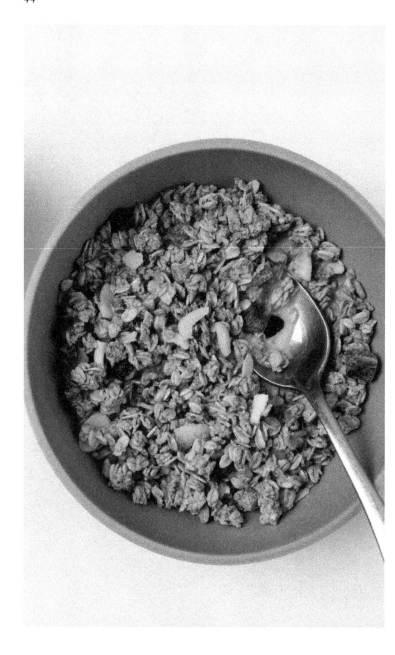

WATER

Even on the water was felt everything. Let's be clear.

Our body is made for the most part of water: about 70%, with percentages that vary according to age (generally the quantity decreasing with the passing of the years). The water is lost daily through sweating or urinating, so we have to drink things to restore body fluids. The importance of staying well hydrated is fundamental for all chemical processes in the body, both during any time of the day and during physical activity. The amount of water is closely related to calorie consumption: we talk about one liter of water for every thousand calories, or 30 deciliters for every 10 kilos. It follows that consumption can never be the same every day: there is the day when you will train intensively and you will have to drink much more. Do not exaggerate or force yourself: the 2 liters of water required per day, which has been mentioned so many times, are not covered anywhere.

Yes, you can use water to lose weight using it in a strategic way: drinking two glasses of water before eating gives a greater sense of satiety. With a lemon squeezed inside, even better.

CONDIMENTS

Seasonings are raw materials to be chosen with care. Cold-pressed animal fats and vegetable oils are necessary for health: they provide energy, promote the absorption of fat-soluble vitamins (A, D, E and K) and carotenoids, protect nerves and brain, nourish the skin and keep it elastic. But maintaining control is very, very difficult: how many times have we poured oil into the salad in a rain shower? That oil, although it doesn't look like it, will end up weighing in the daily caloric count. But condiments are not only fat, there are low calorie, or even zero calories, that can give flavor without making us accumulate fat.

To avoid are, with no doubt, those of animal origin: butter, cream, lard, from a nutritional point of view have a high content of saturated fatty acids that tend to raise cholesterol levels, as well as coconut and palm vegetable oils.

Vegetable fats (cold pressed olive oil and oilseeds in general) with a high content of unsaturated fatty acids, which do not raise cholesterol and, depending on the type, can even counteract its formation, should be preferred. But be careful, a single teaspoon is 90-100 kcal.

Finally, the best condiments: herbs and spices, vinegar and lemon juice. Practically zero calories and multipurpose.

GREEN

The insufficiency or total lack of vegetables is one of the most serious mistakes that can be made in a diet.

NEVER skimp on vegetables! Vegetables have a high water content (from 75% to 95% by weight), while carbohydrates, proteins and lipids are present in small quantities.

The contribution made by them to reach the daily energy quota is negligible, but here, as for other foods we've seen, they have their strong point in satiating power: a plate of salad before every meal, also based on carbohydrates, helps to fill the stomach and make us avoid the encore (always paying attention to seasonings, of course).

The primary importance of vegetables comes from their vitamin-mineral intake. However, they must be chosen carefully: it's not enough to eat them in quantity to satisfy the daily needs of all vitamins and minerals.

For instance:

the intake of B vitamins, apart from asparagus, is almost completely inconsistent. Vitamin C, is present in low quantities in some vegetables while in others it is very high. Some vegetables such as carrots, spinach, lettuce, radicchio, celery are instead rich in carotenes (carotenoids) precursors of vitamin A: in practice they allow our body to "build" this vitamin. These substances also seem to have an important role in the prevention of certain types of cancer and some chronic diseases due to their antioxidant properties.

As far as minerals are concerned, normally leafy vegetables represent a good source of calcium and iron, however, as they are found associated with other substances, they are little used by our body.

In vegetables, especially leafy vegetables, we also find essential trace elements such as manganese, copper, zinc, very important for our body. Some have protective antioxidant action, others are constituents of cell membranes, many enzymes and intervene in the metabolism of carbohydrates, proteins and lipids.

Another important element is the fiber content, which we talked about earlier separately.

In short, yes to vegetables, in all meals, of all colors!

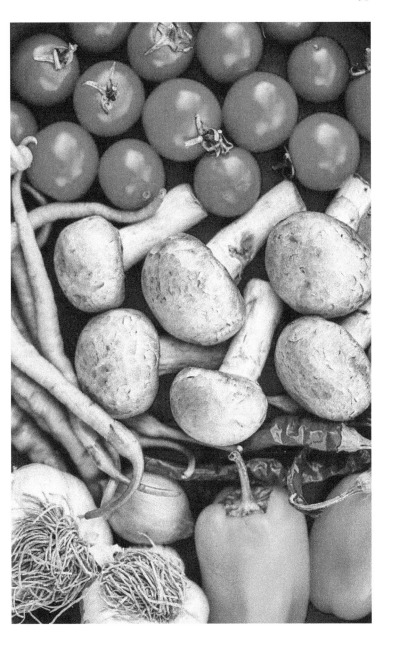

WHOLE SUGARS

What is sugar actually good for?

For a long time it was heard that sugar was essential to support muscle activity or brain function and so on. It's not technically wrong: when doing physical activity, the muscle needs glucose to optimize performance, especially at a certain intensity; and the brain is undoubtedly an organ that consumes a lot of energy in general and sugar in particular. However, what wasn't said is that the sugars that serve the muscles and the brain the body produces on its own from more complex foods that are not necessarily sweets, snacks, soft drinks and so on, but fruit, vegetables and whole grains. There has been, therefore, a distorted interpretation of technically true information.

Actually, the real sugars in the daily diet do not have any metabolic value, but they support only one thing: the palate. They are good, they are tasty, they are satisfying and give a sense of satisfaction. It is no coincidence that when you have moments of discouragement, if you are sweet at home the temptation to throw yourself into them without restraint is very strong. This has been the big trap for the vast majority of people. In the past centuries, in fact, such foods were very rare on the tables of ordinary people, both for processing and cost. During the last century, with the advent of the industrialization of food (and at the same time a consequent drop in quality) and with a cunning market research that has identified sugar as a dependency factor, sugar has become an integral part of, practically, every kind of food. Going to the supermarket and reading the labels, it is really hard to find foods that don't have added sugar.

This combination of two factors, namely the presence on the market of a huge amount of foods with sugar and our tendency to use these foods to compensate for the negative aspects of our lives, has created an explosive mixture. In a country like the USA, the summa of Western prosperity, you can consume up to 70 kg of sugar per person per year. In Italy, although we aren't at these levels, we're still above what would be necessary. If we then add to this aspect the fact that the vast majority of the cereals we consume (pasta, bread, rice, pizza) are refined, then the fiber is removed and therefore have a function within our body that if we do not deviate so much from sugar, and add to all this food such as snacks, various sweets, sugary drinks, comes out a quantity of sugar load really above our metabolic capacity.

 So, what does this involve? A whole series of very serious problems, often grouped under the name of "diseases of well-being". If there is in fact a single thing we could avoid doing to improve our eating habits, it would be to eliminate sugars from our daily diet and eat cereals in quantities that vary according to physical activity, always 100% whole wheat.

Refined sugar is an accelerator of aging through a process called glycation; it increases insulin levels which leads to an increased risk of cardiometabolic disease and probably also of some cancers. Therefore, besides being a nutritionally almost useless food, it is also potentially harmful.

This does not mean that it should be 100% eliminated, that every cake should be demonized as the absolute evil. It is all a matter of daily habits that must become exceptions. Even once every six months at McDonald's (and that stuff has a scary sugar load) is not something that kills us. If the sugar is whole wheat, even better. One must always gratify oneself: enjoy the exception without guilt within a regulated regime.

MEAT and FISH

Meat or fish? White meat or red meat?

Let's make a premise: as we said before, we divide them between animals and plants but our organism does not make this difference. If we eat good vegetable proteins, matching them with each other is fine, even if their biological value is not optimal.

Having said that, we emphasize one factor: QUALITY.

We are interested to know 1) where the meat-fish comes from 2) how the animal was raised 3) what kind of feed it was given. It often happens, to people who do not control what they buy, to eat too salty food with too many preservatives that have been subjected to antibiotics and also too many saturated fats of poor quality. Sliced meats and sausages, for example, from this point of view only deleterious: they are meats that have undergone a lot of processing and are full of preservatives, not to mention that the WHO has classified them as potentially carcinogenic. It's hard, because they are tasty foods, but if we want to do ourselves a favor we should eliminate them from our diet forever. Then, we can say that a chicken reared according to organic criteria, so outdoors and in fairly large spaces, is undoubtedly better than one reared in batteries. The meat of a Chianina breed cow, grazed according to different standards, is undoubtedly better than normal meat from intensive farming. A fish caught at sea is much better than a farmed fish (the difference can be seen much in salmon, for example). You have to pay a lot of attention to all this and also be willing to spend a little bit more, sometimes a lot more. Our health depends on it.

Better white or red meat?

The color of the meat is due to myoglobin, a protein present in the muscles of animals that allows them to incorporate oxygen to support muscle effort. The color of the meat therefore depends on the different amount of myoglobin contained: the meat with higher amounts of myoglobin are red, those that contain less are white or less red. The more the muscular effort of the animal is sustained (beef, horse, etc.) the more red the meat becomes.

At the protein level the differences are almost zero, both have the same amount. The difference lies in the intake of lipids and minerals: white meats are notoriously leaner, with less saturated fat and less cholesterol. On the other hand, white meat has less iron.

Definitely, it's usually recommended to consume more white meat than red during the week, because white meat is leaner and the intake of noble proteins is essentially the same. Especially if you have cholesterol and cardiovascular problems and in low-calorie diets, white meat is preferable.

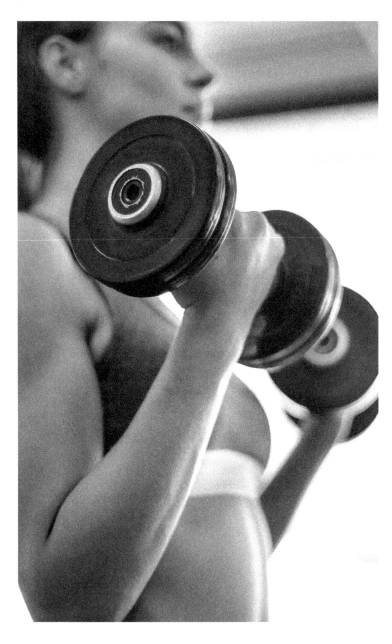

MANAGE MEALS ACCORDING TO YOUR INCLINATIONS

Don't trust who say "absolutely 5 meals a day", "breakfast is always mandatory", "skipping meals lowers the metabolism and raises the cortisol".

What is metabolism? From several factors.

We have the basal metabolism, that is all the internal processes of our body, so the energy that the body consumes only to stay still, in practice; then we have the lifestyle, the work activity, the sport activity that must affect how much we consume and finally also what we eat can affect the total metabolism.

10% of the daily caloric expenditure is given by how much we consume in digesting and assimilating food. As mentioned before, protein is the macronutrient that most needs energy to be broken down and assimilated (about a quarter of total calories). So, when they say that not eating lowers the metabolism is simply because this energy expenditure to absorb food disappears.

In a person who has become accustomed to fasting for a few hours, the hormones antagonistic to insulin are activated in his body; the sympathetic system (the one that keeps us awake) increases at the expense of the parasympathetic system; it is true that cortisol also rises, but it has a lipolytic action (mobilizes fat reserves).

So we can say that it all boils down to a habit: if we used to eat twice a day, we will be hungry twice a day; five times, five times hungry a day. Fasting periods of up to 18 hours brings an increase in insulin sensitivity so with the same carbohydrates the insulin will rise less and we'll have a caloric partitioning towards the muscle and not only towards the fat.

Finally, the discriminating factor is the amount of calories we ingest through food that determines how much we spend to assimilate it. The number of meals is irrelevant, so adjust yourself to how you feel.

PLANS

Let's now see some examples on how to deal with an effective slimming system. Let's be clear: everything I have written so far is the basis for any type of diet that lasts over time. There are no secrets or magic formulas, as already explained: it is all about respecting those certain parameters, knowing what you are eating and using tricks to limit the sense of hunger.

First of all, you have to calculate the daily calorie requirement. To do so, just one of the many apps that can be found, even free of charge, on the various stores. Then, calculate an amount of calories about 25% less the first week (more impactful) and 15-20% less the following weeks.

In the first week, in fact, you have to take advantage of the psychological motivation to shake up the metabolism and you can then deviate from the perfect partition of macronutrients giving priority to proteins and reducing carbohydrates and lipids.

Remember: there is no other way to have control over what you eat than by counting CALORIES. Those who say "eat as much of that food as you want" say a fregnaccia, because even if it was protein, so with 25 calories out of 100 burned to digest them, the other 75 are there and count.

This first week will therefore be based on:
- fish
- white meat
- eggs
- Red meat as lean as possible and of high quality (better if undercooked or raw)
- vegetables
- legumes

So let's delete the foods richer in carbohydrates and fats: we do not zero them, however, because vegetable proteins (beans, lentils, chickpeas, tofu) also have a good amount of carbohydrates. Zeroing a macronutrient as they want the most aggressive low carb diets (such as Dukan or ketogenic) brings a greater immediate weight loss, but just two weeks of this regime and the hunger impulse will manifest itself with such violence that it is almost impossible to resist (and we will have there cells and enzymes with their receptors stretched to the maximum ready to metabolize every single molecule, so as to put back on more fat than before).

In the following weeks we will return to add sugar-rich foods such as bread or pasta (ALWAYS wholemeal) and fruit. The important thing will be, as usual, to count the heat. The calorie intake will have to be increasing over time: in the second week we will have one day with a normal calorie intake, in the third week two days, in the fourth three days and so on. When you reach a stalemate, i.e. a point where you realize you are no longer losing weight, start this cycle again from the beginning.

For the rest, just apply the small rules and strategies that I have listed, many bricks that go to build a regular regime: eliminate everything that, besides being of little nutritional value, is potentially harmful (cold cuts, sausages, industrial sweets, carbonated drinks); remember to be hyper-parsimonious with condiments; remember to drink a glass of water before eating, as well as vegetables; drink green tea and coffee, better if not sweetened, given their thermogenic power; and above all, do a lot of exercise, of different types (both aerobic, which burns mostly fat, and anaerobic, which burns mostly carbohydrates) as regularly as possible.

If you follow all these rules the results will not be long in coming.

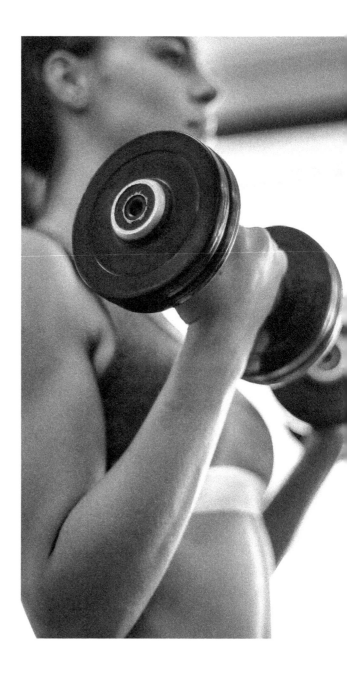

WEEKLY PROGRAM

WEEKLY PLAN FOR THE FIRST WEEK

We now see a plan suitable for the first week of our diet, a partial discharge of carbohydrates and lipids combined with a low-calorie regime. This model will then be replicated in the following weeks by introducing, on alternate days, a regular caloric day (first week none, second week on Sunday, third week on Wednesday and Sunday and so on) where we can eat pasta or rice (wholemeal) or even a piece of chocolate, until we reach a stalemate. When you are no longer able to get down in weight, start again.

Monday

Breakfast:

- coffee (note: as I have already said, with a view to managing meals according to one's inclinations, I found it rewarding on morning training to drink exclusively a coffee with a teaspoon of sugar. If instead you are used to having breakfast, add a toast with 0 sugar jam)

Lunch:

- beans (good protein content combined with carbohydrates)
- mixed leaf salad seasoned with lemon, vinegar and a tablespoon of oil (before beans)

Dinner:

- meat tartare seasoned with salt, pepper, a tablespoon of oil, lemon, capers, onion and egg
- carrots

Tuesday

Breakfast:
- coffee

Lunch:
- stewed lentils
- mixed leaf salad seasoned with lemon, vinegar and a tablespoon of oil (before lentils)

Dinner:
- Pan-fried salmon with Philadelphia light and chives
- Raw fennel

Wednesday

Breakfast:
- coffee

Lunch:
- seitan steak
- mixed leaf salad seasoned with lemon, vinegar and a tablespoon of oil (before seitan)

Dinner:
- Chicken with lemon, ginger and soya sauce
- broccoli

Thursday

Breakfast:

- coffee

Lunch:

- cannellini beans all'uccelletto
- mixed leaf salad seasoned with lemon, vinegar and a tablespoon of oil (before seitan)

Dinner:

- salad meat in carpaccio, arugula and Grana cheese

Friday

Breakfast:
- coffee

Lunch:
- chickpeas and rosemary
- mixed leaf salad seasoned with lemon, vinegar and a tablespoon of oil (before seitan)

Dinner:
- Chianina burger with tabasco sauce
- Boiled potatoes and parsley

Saturday

Breakfast:
- coffee

Lunch:
- barley soup without bacon
- mixed leaf salad seasoned with lemon, vinegar and a tablespoon of oil (before the soup)

Dinner:
- Boiled eggs
- Asparagus

Sunday

Breakfast:
- coffee

Lunch:
- white sponge beans in tomato sauce
- mixed leaf salad seasoned with lemon, vinegar and a tablespoon of oil (before beans)

Dinner:
- Saffron shrimps
- Fennel

And remember: this diet has been set to guarantee the most limited food sacrifice, but if you don't feel the hunger bites increase in any way, it means you are not losing weight. Reduce the portions or reduce the seasonings.

CPSIA information can be obtained
at www.ICGtesting.com
Printed in the USA
BVHW012059250321
603178BV00034B/453